INSULIN
RESISTANCE

The Complete Guide to Reverse Insulin
Resistance & Manage Weight

Donald A. Thomas

Table of Contents

CHAPTER 1

WHAT IS INSULIN RESISTANCE?

Insulin resistance, similarly known as harmed insulin diploma of stage of sensitivity, takes place whilst cells for your muscular tissue mass, fats and liver don`t reply as they need to to insulin, a hormone consultant your pancreatic makes this is important absolutely and controling blood sugar stage (sugar) tiers. Insulin resistance can doubtlessly be transient or constant and is treatable in loads of cases.

Under recurring situations, insulin runs within side the sticking to activities:

Your frame troubles down the meals you are taking in into sugar (sugar) that is your frame's principal supply of electricity.

Sugar enters your blood move, which suggests your pancreatic to launch insulin.

Insulin allows sugar for your blood input into your muscular tissue mass, fats and liver cells that will doubtlessly use it for electricity or watch for withinside the destiny use.

When sugar enters your cells and the tiers for your blood move decrease, it suggests your pancreatic to save you growing insulin.

For loads of aspects, your muscular tissue mass, fats and liver cells can doubtlessly reply incorrectly to insulin, which recommends they can not correctly inhabit sugar out of your blood or wait. This is insulin resistance. As a result, your pancreatic makes greater insulin to goal to achieve over your enhancing blood sugar stage tiers. This is known as hyperinsulinemia.

As large as your pancreatic can doubtlessly make ok insulin to achieve over your cells' vulnerable reactions to insulin, your blood sugar tiers will clearly really stay in a healthful and balanced in addition to stabilized differ. If your cells wound up being additionally unsusceptible to insulin, it result in accelerated blood sugar stage tiers (hyperglycemia), which, in time, result in prediabetes and Type 2 diabetic troubles mellitus.

Together with Type 2 diabetic troubles mellitus, insulin resistance pertains to loads of oneof-a-kind numerous different troubles, containing:

- Extreme weight.

- Cardiovascular disease.

- Nonalcoholic fatty liver problem.

- Metabolic situation.

- Polycystic ovary situation (PCOS).

What is the distinction among insulin resistance and diabetic troubles mellitus?

Anyone can doubtlessly produce insulin resistance — quick

or persistantly. In time, constant insulin resistance can doubtlessly cause prediabetes in addition to later on Type 2 diabetic troubles mellitus if it is now no longer controlled or capable of be controlled.

Prediabetes takes place whilst your blood sugar stage tiers are extra than recurring, but decreased ok to be located as diabetic troubles mellitus. Prediabetes commonly happens in human beings that currently have a few insulin resistances.

Prediabetes can doubtlessly cause Type 2 diabetic troubles

mellitus (T2D), amongst one of the maximum regular form of diabetic troubles mellitus. T2D takes place whilst your pancreatic would not make ok insulin or your frame would not use insulin properly (insulin resistance), inflicting excessive blood sugar stage tiers.

Type 1 diabetic troubles mellitus (T1D) takes place whilst your frame's frame frame immune device moves and troubles the insulin-generating cells for your pancreatic for an unidentified variable. T1D is an autoimmune and constant problem, and those with T1D must instill fabricated insulin to real-time and be healthful and balanced in addition to stabilized. While T1D isn't prompt via way of means of insulin resistance, human beings with T1D can doubtlessly enjoy tiers of insulin resistance wherein their cells do not reply properly to the insulin they instill.

Gestational diabetic troubles mellitus is a temporary create of diabetic troubles mellitus that may doubtlessly manifest even as expectant. It's prompt via way of means of insulin resistance this is consequently of the hormone representatives the placenta makes. Gestational diabetic troubles mellitus vanishes whilst you provide your baby. About three% to 8% of anybody who're looking forward to human beings within side the Combined Defines are located with gestational diabetic troubles mellitus.

Medical expert regularly use a blood assessment known as glycated hemoglobin (A1C) to decide diabetic troubles mellitus. It packages your not unusual place blood sugar stage for the preceding three months. Usually:

An A1C stage indexed right here 5.7% is concept of recurring.

An A1C stage among 5.7% and 6.four% is concept of prediabetes.

An A1c stage of 6.5% or better on 2 numerous exams recommends kind 2 diabetic troubles mellitus.

People with Type 1 diabetic troubles mellitus commonly have an certainly excessive A1C and relatively excessive blood sugar stage tiers after medical scientific analysis because of that their pancreatic is growing bit or no insulin.

Insulin resistance can doubtlessly have an effect on anyone — you do not must have diabetic troubles mellitus — and it may doubtlessly be transient (as an example, using steroid medicine for a quick duration develops insulin resistance) or constant. Both principal sides that display as much as consist of in insulin resistance is extra frame fats, particularly concerning your continual stomach, and a loss of workout.

People which have prediabetes and Type 2 diabetic

troubles mellitus commonly have a few stage of insulin resistance. People with Type 1 diabetic troubles mellitus can doubtlessly similarly enjoy insulin resistance.

Since there commonly are not any form of form of regular exams to searching out insulin resistance and there commonly are not any form of form of signs up until it turns into prediabetes or Type 2 diabetic troubles mellitus, one of the maximum dependable implies to pick out the occasion of insulin resistance is the use of the choice of prediabetes circumstances. Higher than eighty four million grownups within side the Combined Defines have prediabetes. That's traumatic 1 from each three grownups

Specifically simply how does insulin resistance have an effect on my frame?

The improvement of insulin resistance generally boosts insulin production (hyperinsulinemia) so your frame can doubtlessly preserve healthful and balanced in addition to stabilized blood sugar tiers. Increased tiers of insulin can doubtlessly result in weight get, which, as a result, makes insulin resistance additionally even worse.

Hyperinsulinemia is similarly related to the sticking to troubles:

- Higher triglyceride tiers.
- Hardening of the arteries (atherosclerosis).
- Hypertension (hypertension).

Insulin resistance is similarly the emphasize of metabolic situation, that is a group of connects that net net hyperlink extra fats concerning the waistline and insulin resistance to accelerated danger of cardiovascular disease, stroke and Type 2 diabetic troubles mellitus.

Connects of metabolic situation contain:

- Increased blood sugar stage tiers.
- An accelerated triglyceride stage.
- Minimized tiers of excessive-density lipoprotein (HDL) cholesterol.
- Hypertension.

You do not must have all four of those connects to have metabolic situation.

What are the signs of? Obtained elements for insulin resistance

Obtained develops, displaying you're now no longer birthed with the purpose, of insulin resistance contain:

Added frame fats: Scientists expect intense weight, mainly delivered fats to your chronic belly in addition to concerning your frame frame organs (all-herbal fats), is a essential starting place aid of insulin resistance. A waistline size of forty inches or greater for people in addition to humans marked man at delivery in addition to 35 inches or greater for ladies in addition to humans marked women at delivery is related to insulin resistance. Research look at seems into have in reality disclosed that chronic belly fats makes hormone representatives in addition to several diverse different materials which can make contributions to resilient swelling to your frame. This swelling may upload in insulin resistance

Physical absence of exercise: Workout makes your frame greater conscious insulin in addition to constructs muscular tissues mass which can soak up blood glucose. An loss of exercise will have in reality opposite outcomes in addition to purpose insulin resistance. Moreover, an loss of exercise in addition to a miles much less lively manner of residing are pertains to weight get, that can moreover make contributions to insulin resistance.

Diet routine strategy: A weight loss plan routine recurring of particularly fine-tuned, excessive-carbohydrate ingredients in addition to loaded fat become related to insulin resistance. Your frame digests particularly fine-tuned, excessive-carbohydrate ingredients particularly immediately, which produces your blood sugar to rise. This regions greater anxiety and additionally strain and nervousness to your pancreatic to create a big quantity of insulin, which, in time, can cause insulin resistance.

Specific medicinal drugs: Specific medicinal drugs can purpose insulin resistance, containing steroids, a few high blood pressure medicinal drugs, and precise HIV remedies in addition to a few intellectual medicinal drugs.

Your frame makes diverse hormone representatives, which can be chemical compounds that crew up severa runs to your frame via way of means of lugging messages thru your blood for frame organs, muscular tissues mass in addition to several diverse different cells. These suggests notify your frame what to do whilst to do it.

Troubles with precise hormone representatives can have an effect on exactly precisely how properly your frame uses insulin. Hormonal agent problems which can purpose insulin resistance consist of:

Cushing's trouble: This hassle takes place whilst there is greater cortical to your frame. Cortisol, the "anxiety and additionally strain and nervousness hormone representative," is crucial to controlling your blood sugar tiers (via way of means of boosting them) in addition to converting meals into power. Added cortisol can counteract the outcomes of insulin, triggering insulin resistance.

Acromegaly: This is an unusual but intense hassle that takes place if you have in reality excessive tiers of development hormone representative (GH). High tiers of GH can purpose stepped forward manufacturing of sugar that can cause insulin resistance.

Hypothyroidism: This hassle takes place whilst your thyroid is underactive in addition to would not create good enough thyroid hormone representative. Your thyroid performs a large paintings in controling your metabolic price (exactly precisely how your frame changes the meals you consume into power). When it makes insufficient thyroid hormone representative, containing your sugar metabolic price that can purpose insulin resistance.

Genetic problems that broaden insulin resistance

Particular were given genetic problems (problems you are birthed with) can broaden insulin resistance for diverse factors.

There's a set of uncommon pertinent problems defined as were given excessive insulin resistance syndromes which can be taken into consideration detail of a vary. Kept in thoughts from numerous modest to numerous excessive, those syndromes consist of:

Type an insulin resistance trouble: In humans with Type A insulin resistance trouble, insulin resistance damages blood glucose diploma law in addition to truly purpose diabetes mellitus. The insulin resistance in addition to several diverse different signs usually does not get up up until teenage years or later. It's usually now no longer hazardous.

People which have actually trouble are abnormally little beginning within side the preceding delivery, in addition to harmed babies enjoy cannot prosper, which suggests they do not develop in addition to area on weight on the predicted cost. People with trouble broaden symptoms and symptoms and additionally signs definitely very early in existence in addition to on line into their teens or 20s. Casualty usually broadens from problems linked with diabetes mellitus.

Donohue trouble: People with Donohue trouble are abnormally little beginning within side the preceding delivery, in addition to harmed babies enjoys cannot prosper. Added signs that get up now no longer prolonged after delivery consist of an loss of cellulite below the skin, throwing out (deterioration) of muscle cells in addition to manner an excessive amount of frame hair development (hirsutism). Several kids with this hassle do poor thru preceding age 2.

Miltonic dystrophy: This is a type of muscular tissues dystrophy that impacts your muscle cells, eyes in addition to endocrine gadget frame frame organs, that includes your pancreatic. Muscle cells insulin diploma of stage of sensitivity is decreased via way of means of annoying 70% in humans with myotonic dystrophy, which purpose insulin resistance.

Alström trouble: This is an uncommon were given hassle that is decided via way of means of a current lack of imaginative and prescient in addition to hearing, broadened cardiomyopathy, weight problems, Type 2 diabetes mellitus mellitus in addition to brief stature.

Werner trouble: This is an uncommon colorful hassle that is decided via way of means of the arrival of abnormally quickened maturing (progeria). It impacts several additives of your frame, containing unusual manufacturing of insulin in addition to resistance to the outcomes of insulin.

Got lipodystrophy: This is an trouble wherein your frame would not employ in addition to hold fats suitably. The enormous starting place aid of insulin resistance in lip dystrophy is that unwanted sugar cannot be conserved in fats cells.

Exactly how is insulin resistance discovered?

Insulin resistance is hard to decide because of that there is not definitely clearly everyday trying out for it, in addition to as extended as your pancreatic is generating good enough insulin to achieve over the resistance, you'll now no longer have in reality any type of form of signs.

As there is no solitary examination which can immediately decide insulin resistance, your healthcare answer commercial enterprise will definitely recollect a whole lot of factors whilst comparing insulin resistance, containing your:

- Scientific history.
- House history.
- Physical examination.
- Signs and additionally signs.
- Exam results.

What critiques will definitely be carried out to take a look

Slowly, that manner of dwelling adjustments can:

Enhance insulin diploma of stage of sensitivity (lessen insulin resistance).

Reduce high blood pressure.

Reduce triglyceride in addition to LDL ("inadequate") ldl cholesterol tiers.

Boost HDL ("fantastic") ldl cholesterol tiers.

You may manage severa numerous different scientific professional, inclusive of a nutritional professional in addition to endocrinologist, similarly in your ordinary doctor to increase an individualized remedy method that operates largest for you.

What drugs are made use to address insulin resistance?

While there are presently no drugs that manage insulin resistance mainly, your healthcare answer commercial enterprise may recommend drugs to address coexisting issues. Some situations include:

- Hypertension medication

- Metformin for diabetes

mellitus mellitus.

- Statins to decrease LDL ldl cholesterol.

Can I opposite insulin resistance?

Insulin resistance has genuinely a lot of produces in addition to together with elements. While manner of dwelling adjustments, inclusive of ingesting a healthful and balanced and additionally stabilized food plan routine, exercise regularly in addition to dropping unwanted weight, can decorate insulin diploma of stage of sensitivity in addition to lessen insulin resistance, now no longer all produces are fairly very clean to take care of.

Talk you your healthcare answer commercial enterprise disturbing what you may do to largest control insulin resistance.

Your weight loss plan application has a large end result to your blood glucose diploma in addition to insulin tiers. Extremely improved, excessive-carbohydrate in addition to excessive-fats meals require greater insulin.

All at once, ingesting meals which have in reality a minimized to tool glycemic index in addition to proscribing meals which have in reality a excessive glycemic index will sincerely useful resource you opposite in addition to/or address insulin resistance. Eating meals with fiber additionally allows manage blood glucose diploma tiers due to that it takes your frame plenty longer to take in fiber, displaying your blood glucose diploma tiers don`t upward thrust as a terrific deal.

The glycemic index (GI) is a dimension that positions meals having genuinely carbohydrates inning conformity with in reality what does it set you back? they impact your blood glucose diploma tiers. The Glycemic Index Framework (GIF) classifies the GI of meals as both minimized, tool or excessive, with natural sugar generally as a advice at 100:

Minimized GI: fifty five or plenty a good deal much less.

Device GI: 56-69.

High GI: 70 or greater

High-GI meals generally have in reality lots of carbohydrates in addition to/or sugar in addition to minimized to no fiber net net content. Low-GI meals generally have in reality minimized quantities of carbohydrates in addition to better quantities of fiber.

- White bread.
- Potatoes.
- Breakfast cereals.
- Cakes in addition to cookies.
- Fruits inclusive of

watermelo
n in
addition to
days.

- Beans in addition to legumes.
- Fruits inclusive of apples in addition to berries.
- Non-starchy veggies, inclusive of

asparagus, cauliflower in addition to leafed environment-friendliness.

Nuts.

- Milk, fish in addition to meat.

Frequently chat together along with your healthcare answer commercial enterprise within side the preceding production excessive modifications for a food plan routine application.

What are the hazard aspects for growing insulin resistance?

Certain genetic in addition to way of life hazard aspects make it greater than possibly that you may sincerely increase insulin resistance or prediabetes. Risk aspects include:

Overweight or weight issues, mainly unwanted fats regarding your tummy.

Being age forty five or older.

A first-diploma favored one (mamas in addition to papa or bro or sis) with diabetes mellitus mellitus.

Having genuinely in reality a miles much less active way of life.
Certain fitness and health in addition to fitness issues, inclusive of high blood pressure in addition to unusual ldl cholesterol tiers.

Records of gestational diabetes mellitus mellitus.

Records of coronary heart trouble or stroke.

Having genuinely in reality a calming trouble, inclusive of the rest apnea.

Smoking cigarettes.

Individuals of the abiding via way of means of racial or ethnic backgrounds also are at a better hazard of getting genuinely in reality insulin resistance or prediabetes:

- Oriental American.
- Black.
- Hispanic/Latino.
- Indigenous people from Alaska.

Indigenous people from the continental Linked Mentions.

Indigenous people from the Pacific Islands.

Although you cannot extrude positive hazard aspects for insulin resistance, inclusive of domestic records or age, you may virtually attempt lowering your probabilities of growing it via way of means of keeping a healthful and balanced in addition to stabilized weight, ingesting a healthful and balanced in addition to stabilized weight loss plan application in addition to exercise regularly.

What is the prognosis (assumption) for insulin resistance?

The prognosis (assumption) of insulin resistance is based on a lot of aspects, containing:

- The starting place useful resource of insulin resistance.
- The energy of insulin resistance.

Exactly how nicely your insulin-generating cells are performance.

Exactly how at hazard you're to growing issues from insulin resistance.

Adherence to remedy in addition to your frame's hobby to remedy.

Individuals can virtually have in reality modest insulin resistance that in no way ever earlier than will become prediabetes or Type 2 diabetes mellitus mellitus. Individuals can virtually additionally have in reality insulin resistance that is fairly easy to restore or exceptionally possible with way of life modifications. For plenty of human beings which have genuinely actually received issues that increase intense insulin resistance, it is able to virtually threaten or purpose death.

If you've got genuinely in reality insulin resistance, ask your healthcare answer commercial enterprise disturbing what you may virtually put together for in addition to precisely how largest to address it.

A lot of the issues that may virtually arise from insulin resistance are associated with the improvement of vascular (blood vessel) issues because of increased blood glucose diploma tiers in addition to increased insulin tiers (hyperinsulinemia).

Not everybody that has insulin resistance will sincerely honestly have in reality issues. If you've got got genuinely been discovered with insulin resistance, Type 2 diabetes mellitus mellitus or metabolic problem, it is crucial to look your healthcare answer commercial enterprise regularly in addition to keep on with your remedy technique to try and live clean of those issues.

When ought to I see my healthcare answer commercial enterprise disturbing insulin resistance?

If you've got genuinely been discovered with insulin resistance or issues associated with insulin resistance, it is crucial to look your healthcare answer commercial enterprise regularly to make certain your blood glucose diploma tiers stay in a healthful and balanced in addition to stabilized fluctuate which your remedy is performance.

If you are experiencing signs of excessive blood glucose diploma or prediabetes, telecellsmartphone name your healthcare answer commercial enterprise.

CHAPTER 2

DIET PLAN POINTERS FOR INSULIN RESISTANCE

Diet plan software guidelines

Typically, it`s best to preference entire, unprocessed meals in addition to continue to be unfastened from fairly progressed in addition to ready meals.

Foods which are fairly progressed, which includes white breads, pastas, rice, in addition to smooth consume, take in fairly quick in addition to can without a doubt beautify blood glucose diploma degrees. These places brought pressure at the pancreatic that makes the hormone consultant insulin.

Your frame is blocking off the insulin from overall performance certainly to lessen blood glucose diploma degrees for folks that are insulin immune.

Loaded fat have honestly moreover been related to insulin resistance. Healthy and balanced in addition to stabilized, unsaturated fat, which includes the ones endorsed under, are a far a good deal a ways better alternative

.   Eating excessive-fiber meals in addition to blended recipes, now no longer simply carbohydrates alone, can without a doubt assist slow-shifting meals digestion in addition to take anxiety off the pancreatic.

Correct indexed under are a few meals which can blend in addition to in shape to assemble pleasurable healthful and balanced in addition to stabilized dishes for any sort of kind of recipe.

Veggies are minimized in energy in addition to excessive in fiber, production them an wonderful meals that will help you address your blood glucose diploma. One of the maximum dependable veggie choices are:

- clean
- low-sodium tinned
- icy

Healthy and balanced in addition to stabilized choices include:

- tomatoes
- asparagus
- inexperienced beans
- carrots

- shiny
  peppers
- eco-
  friendlies
  which
  includes
  spinach,
  collards,
  cabbage in
  addition to
  kale
- cruciferous
  greens
  which
  includes
  broccoli,
  cauliflower
  ,   in

addition to
Brussels
sprouts

Veggie juices can display up healthful and balanced in addition to stabilized, but they have got honestly the propensity to be now no longer as oral dental filling in addition to generally commonly are not as crude as clean greens.

Munch on a few fruit for:

fiber

vitamins

minerals

Choice clean or icy culmination. Tinned varies without consisted of sugars are amazing moreover, but they do not have honestly the fiber that clean in addition to icy culmination do because the skins are removed.

Select culmination which are better in fiber, which includes:

- apples
- berries
- inexperienced bananas
- grapes
- plums
- peaches

Remain unfastened from fruit juices on account that they are able to without a doubt beautify blood glucose diploma as quick as normal smooth consume. Likewise the unsweetened juices or the ones categorized "no sugar consisted of" are excessive in all-herbal sugars.

Milk

Milk elements you the calcium you have to assist marketplace robust enamel in addition to bones. Choice lessens fats, unsweetened milk in addition to yogurt. Stay clean of entire milk in addition to complete-fats yogurts on account that an excessive consumption of hydrogenated fats, located in animal fat, becomes connected to insulin resistance.

If you are lactose intolerant, strive an unsweetened alternative milk like bolstered soy milk or lactose- unfastened cow's milk choices. Rice in addition to almond milk are moreover alternative milk choices, but they have got honestly minimum healthful and balanced healthful protein or dietary nicely worth.

Whole-grain meals are amazing for people with insulin resistance. They're abundant in:

- vitamins
- fiber
- mineral

Many people count on that keeping off all carbohydrates is wanted to keep diabetic character problems, but healthful and balanced in addition to stabilized, entire, unprocessed carbohydrate reassets are simply a excellent fuelling supply in your frame. Nevertheless, it is nevertheless must manipulate regions of those lots a good deal more healthy choices.

It's crucial to cognizance on choosing healthful and balanced in addition to stabilized, unprocessed grains as prolonged as practical. It's moreover crucial to consume those meals as a blended recipe, with healthful and balanced healthful protein in addition to fats, as those should useful resource you continues to be unfastened from blood glucose diploma spikes.

To accumulate the endorsed quantity of nutrients, select merchandise those listing entire-grain active additives at the start at the mark.

- entire-wheat or stone-floor entire grain
- entire oats in addition to oat dish
- bulgur
- entire-grain corn or corn recipe
- brown rice

- entire-grain barley
- entire rye
- wild rice
- entire farro
- quinoa
- millet
- buckwheat

Beans in addition to legumes

Beans are an excellent supply of fiber. They increase blood sugar degree diploma degrees slowly, that's an ad for people with insulin resistance. Some excellent alternatives are:

- pinto
- lima
- purple in addition to black beans

If you are short in a spark off fashion, tinned beans are wonderful choices to dry out beans. Merely confirm to empty pipes pipelines in addition to smooth tinned beans or preference the "no salt consisted of" alternatives on account that they are able to surely be excessive in salt.

Fish it really is complete of omega-three fats can surely lower your threat of coronary heart disease, a not unusual place problem for people with diabetic character problems. Fish abundant in omega-three contain:

- salmon
- mackerel
- herring
- sardines
- tuna
- rainbow trout

Tilapia, cod, flounders, halibut, in addition to haddock are similarly super for you, but they may be lessening in omega-three on accounts that they may be lessen in complete fats. Shellfish fanatics can surely value:

- lobster
- scallops
- shrimp
- oysters
- clams
- crabs

Nevertheless, much like all meals, restrict fish it really is breaded or deep-fried. If you want to soak up deep-fried fish, confirm that it is geared up in a lots a good deal more healthy oil.

To preserve your chook use healthful and balanced in addition to stabilized, peel in addition to toss the pores and skin. Fowl pores and skin has a good deal greater fats compared to the meat. The appropriate information is is, you may surely put together with the pores and skin on keep moistness in addition to later on eliminates it previously you're taking in it.

Try:

- chook busts
- Cornish hen

- turkey

Numerous different lean healthful and balanced healthful protein

As giant as they may be lean, healthful and balanced healthful protein which includes beef, veal, lamb, in addition to red meat are super when you have honestly virtually insulin resistance. You must truly select out:

- beef tenderloin or middle loin chops

- veal loin chops or roasts
- lamb chops, roasts, or legs
- alternative
- or select out lean red meat with the fats reduced

Ground red meat with lessen fats net cloth is supplied. You can surely preference floor turkey.

Vegan healthful and balanced healthful protein reassets can absolutely be splendid alternatives also. Exceptional options contain:

- soy
- temper
- beans
- tofu
- legumes

Healthy and balanced in addition to stabilized fat

Choice healthful and balanced in addition to stabilized unsaturated fats reasserts. This fat can surely lessen meals digestion in addition to offer essential fats.

Nuts, seeds, in addition to nut in addition to seed butters offer:

- healthful and balanced in addition to stabilized fat
- magnesium
- healthful and balanced healthful protein fiber
- fiber

Nuts in addition to seeds are further reduced in carbohydrates, with a purpose to sincerely profits any type of precise looking to control their blood sugar stage degree.

Heart-healthful omega-three fats are further located in a few nuts in addition to seeds like flax seeds in addition to walnuts. Yet make sure. Nuts, at the same time as fairly healthful and balanced in addition to stabilized, are further excessive in energy. They can surely encompass technique a whole lot of energy for a food regimen routine ordinary if they`re now no longer efficaciously portioned.

Keep in thoughts particularly precisely how nuts in addition to seeds prepare. Some offers with, at the side of nut in addition to seed butters, encompass consisted of salt in addition to sugar. This can honestly beautify the energy in addition to lower the dietary properly really well worth of the nuts or nut butter.

Avocados in addition to olives are further wonderful alternatives. Cooking with olive oil in preference to stable fat is recommended.

Exercise

Regular workout can surely assist prevent diabetic man or woman issues with the aid of using:

- lowering your blood sugar stage degree
- lowering frame fats
- lessening weight

It further enables your cells grow to be extra conscious insulin.

You do not have to finish a triathlon to get fit. Anything that obtains you moving accredits as workout. Do something you fee such as:

- horticulture
- walking
- walking
- swimming
- dancing

Keep moving to lose energy in addition to maintain your blood sugar stage degrees on target. New necessities suggest dividing enjoyable time each 1/2 of human resources.

Likewise in case you are brief in a activate fashion; you could surely easily encompass brief bouts of process into your day.

At the workplace, take the stairways in preference to the increase in addition to walk the block for the duration of your lunch human resources. In your house, play a pc recreation of document together along with your kids or stroll in placement as you admire television. When you are walking jobs, park loads good enough tons out of your region to get an wonderful stroll in.

Exercise gathers — 10 minutes three instances an afternoon overall as much as fifty percentage an hr of task.

Weight loss

Being overweight or obese improves your chance for diabetic man or woman issues in addition to diabetes-associated problems. Nevertheless, losing likewise some delivered more kilos can surely lower your chance for ailment, at the same time as further assisting control your sugar degrees.

A 2002 take a look at uncovered that losing five to 7 percentage of your frame weight should useful resource in reducing your chance for diabetic man or woman issues with the aid of using better than fifty percentage.

Existing follow-up take a look at appears into have uncovered that weight reduction of seven to ten percentage gives perfect evasion of kind 2 diabetic man or woman issues. For example, in case your beginning weight is two hundred delivered more kilos, losing 14 - 20 delivered more kilos will sincerely make an sizeable difference.

One of the maximum green technique to head down weight is

to absorb tons much less energy in comparison to you lose in addition to workout continually on a every day basis.

It's essential to be realistic for your ingesting technique in addition to workout normal. Develop small functions which can be available in addition to precise.

For example, begin with one healthful and balanced in addition to stabilized extrude for a food regimen routine ordinary in addition to one development for a process stage. Remember, slimming down will now no longer show up over evening. Weight loss is lots tons much less made complicated in comparison to retaining that weight reduction lasting. Placing within side the second to construct new way of life strategies is essential.

Several human beings do unknown they have got insulin resistance up until it involves be kind 2 diabetic man or woman issues.

If you are at chance for prediabetes or diabetic man or woman issues, ask your medical doctor to assessment for it. Checking your hemoglobin A1c stage can surely assist well known insulin resistance or prediabetes previously in comparison to a widespread now no longer ingesting blood sugar stage degree.

If you screen insulin resistance extraordinarily very early, you could surely make critical adjustments to lower your chance for generating diabetic man or woman issues in addition to severe well being in addition to fitness problems that may surely characteristic it.

Remember to touch your medical doctor or dietitian previously converting your healthy eating plan ordinary or workout ordinary. They should useful resource you set up a healthful and balanced in addition to stabilized recipe technique in addition to an workout normal that best fits your demands.

THE END

www.ingramcontent.com/pod-product-compliance
Lightning Source LLC
Chambersburg PA
CBHW070817170726
48000CB00018B/1013